TOP
FITNESS
A D V I C E

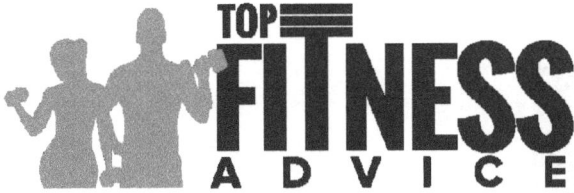

5:2 DIET FOR BEGINNERS

2nd Edition

9 Steps to Lose Weight & Feel Great
On A Fasting Diet – Without
TRYING AT ALL!

LINDA WESTWOOD

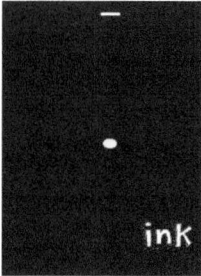

First published in 2015 by Venture Ink Publishing

For more information about the contents of this book or questions to the author, please contact Linda Westwood at linda@topfitnessadvice.com

Disclaimer

This book provides wellness management information in an informative and educational manner only, with information that is general in nature and that is not specific to you, the reader. The contents of this book are intended to assist you and other readers in your personal wellness efforts. Consult your physician regarding the applicability of any information provided in this book to you.

Nothing in this book should be construed as personal advice or diagnosis, and must not be used in this manner. The information provided about conditions is general in nature. This information does not cover all possible uses, actions, precautions, side-effects, or interactions of medicines, or medical procedures. The information in this book should not be considered as complete and does not cover all diseases, ailments, physical conditions, or their treatment.

You should consult with your physician before beginning any exercise, weight loss, or health care program. This book should not be used in place of a call or visit to a competent health-care professional. You should consult a health care professional before adopting any of the suggestions in this book or before drawing inferences from it.

Any decision regarding treatment and medication for your condition should be made with the advice and consultation of a qualified health care professional. If you have, or suspect you have, a health-care problem, then you should immediately contact a qualified health care professional for treatment.

No Warranties: The author and publisher don't guarantee or warrant the quality, accuracy, completeness, timeliness, appropriateness or suitability of the information in this book, or of any product or services referenced in this book.

The information in this book is provided on an "as is" basis and the author and publisher make no representations or warranties of any kind with respect to this information. This book may contain inaccuracies, typographical errors, or other errors.

Table of Contents

Would you prefer to listen to my book, rather than read it?

Download the audiobook version for free!

If you go to the special link below and sign up to Audible as a new customer, you can get the audiobook version of my book completely free.

FAST DIET FOR BEGINNERS

5:2 DIET

9 STEP TO LOSING WEIGHT ON A FASTING DIET

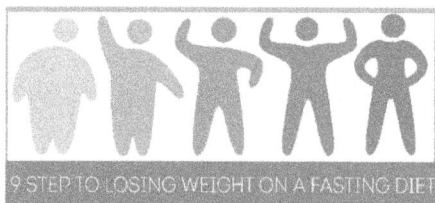

Linda Westwood

"#1 BEST SELLING WEIGHT LOSS AUTHOR"

Go here to get your audiobook version for free:

TopFitnessAdvice.com/go/52diet

Introduction

When you are following a strict diet plan, the most obvious problem that you encounter is what should you actually eat to remain with the diet plan diligently?

To resolve your problems, we are providing you with a few delicious recipes that you can use for your fasting days as well as for non-fasting days.

5:2 diet plan basically decides the amount of calories you are allowed to take in, on each specific day. According to this plan you will never go on a total fast day, but you will just minimize your calorie intake.

To make your each and every day worthwhile, we are giving you recipes with a total of calorie count, so that you can keep a track of calories that you have taken in one meal and thus manage rest of your day accordingly.

Chapter 1

Introduction with 5:2 Diet Plan

Let us start our book with the basic meaning of 5:2 diet plan. According to this diet plan you are supposed to fast for 2 non-consecutive days and have normal and healthy diet for 5 days.

You will need to sustain on 500 calories during these two fasting days but with the kind of diet plan and recipes we have, it is going to be very easy for you. For the rest of the 5 days, you can have 2000 calories per day. Around the world, people are widely accepting this fast diet plan and are quite happy with the output. For men, it is 600 calories and 2500 calories on 2 and 5 days respectively.

We will plan your day in such a way that you take around 100 calories in your breakfast, around 200 in your lunch and under 200 calories for your dinner. This is the way to use your 500 calories in an optimum level. We have breakfast, lunch and dinner recipes for you which will ensure good health and best taste.

Chapter 2

Functioning of 5:2 Diet Plan

5:2 diet plan is another name for intermittent fasting. Fasting is an obvious way of losing fat because you are cutting down on your carbohydrate and fat intake. 5:2 is an efficient way in a sense that you do not go on a long-term starvation mode but you follow a repair mode.

This is a diet plan that works on repairing your damaged cells so that they work in a better way. When you are on starvation mode, you are actually reinforcing your body to store more fat for future use. This method is harmful in a long term. With the help of 5:2 plan you can not only decrease the fat content of your body but also regulate the sugar level of your blood and fight diabetes in a better way.

Discover Scientifically-Proven "Shortcuts" & "Hacks" to Lose Weight FASTER (With Very Little Effort)

For this month only, you can get Linda's best-selling & most popular book absolutely free – *Weight Loss Secrets You NEED to Know*.

Get Your FREE Copy Here:

TopFitnessAdvice.com/Bonus

Discover scientifically-proven tips to help you lose weight faster and easier than ever before. With this book, readers were able to improve their weight loss results and fitness levels. So, it's highly recommended that you get this book, especially while it's free!

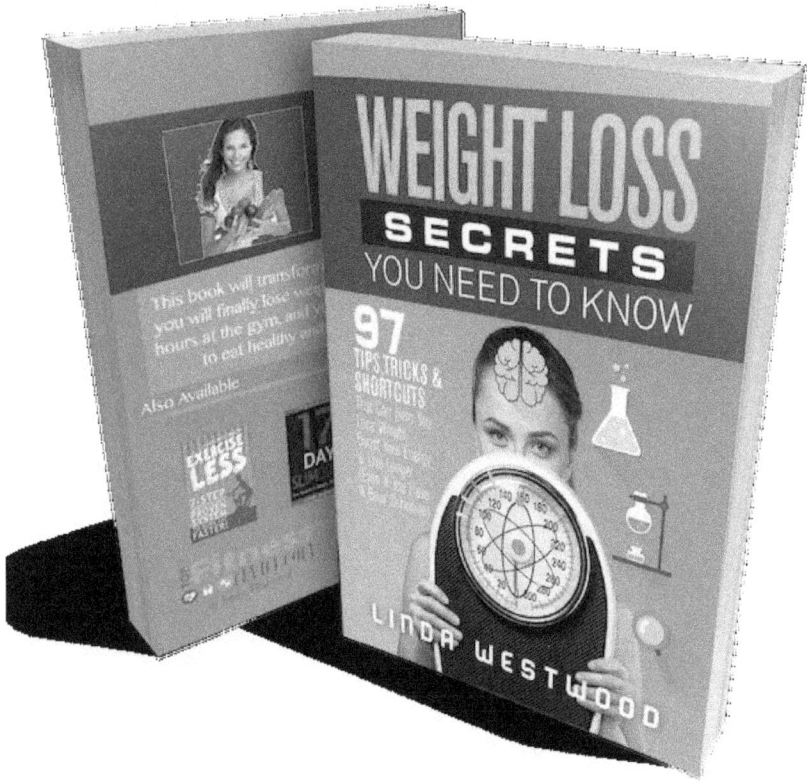

Get Your FREE Copy Here:

TopFitnessAdvice.com/Bonus

Chapter 3

Health Benefits Associated with 5:2 Diet Plan

With a balanced fasting your digestive system will get a rest and it will work longer and in a better way.

With the help of 5:2 diet plan you can change your daily eating habits for good and remain fat free for lifelong. Once you have reduced you have a control on your weight you can fast for one day and maintain a constant weight.
Fasting days might sound difficult but you will get used to this within a few weeks and then you will feel very light for the day without showing any signs of lethargy.

This diet plan reduces your risk of getting any kind of chronic diseases like diabetes type two and more. The diet plan also prohibits the growth of IGF-1 hormone in our body. It is this hormone which accelerates ageing of human body and for some also leads to cancer.

The diet plan is quite simple and flexible and you can continue with this plan for a longer duration because you can enjoy your favorite dishes without feeling guilty about them.

Chapter 4

Precautions and Extra Activities while Following 5:2 Diet Plan

If you are a diabetic patient then before undertaking 5:2 diet you should consult your doctor first. You can also consult a nutritionist and get your diet chart planned with the nutritionist's help. Pregnant women, children and people recovering from injuries should refrain from taking such diets.

If you feel fatigue and energy less in those two fasting days then again consult your doctor before carrying on with the diet plan.

5:2 diet plan is just the initial step towards getting a healthy body. If you want to get faster results, you will need to move a step ahead and do some kind of physical workout. You can start with gym, aerobics or any other form of exercise that suits you.

You should take proper sleep at night so that your metabolism and body clock works perfectly. This is necessary to get healthy results.

If you have any kind of bad habit like smoking and drinking then you should try and change these habits. You should also inculcate the habit of drinking a lot of water on a daily basis. This ensures that all your body waste is excreted out.

In a 5:2 diet plan, it is important to take care of the calorie count during those 5 days. It is easy to miss the target, especially when you have fasted the previous day. If you keep a check on your diet for the rest of non-fasting days, you will witness results within no time.

Chapter 5

2 Days Fasting Recipes for Breakfast and Snacks

You should never skip your breakfast just because you are on a strict diet plan; rather it is important to maintain a balanced diet. You just need to plan your breakfast right.

Devise a diet plan where you can get energy for morning chores and also you intake only 100 calories. We are giving you a few delicious recipes that will suffice your purpose. You can also do a bit of mix and match according to your needs.

If you're enjoying this book and would love to let other potential readers know how great it is, please take a few seconds to leave a review on Amazon.com.

Greek Yogurt, Blueberry Kiwi Smoothie

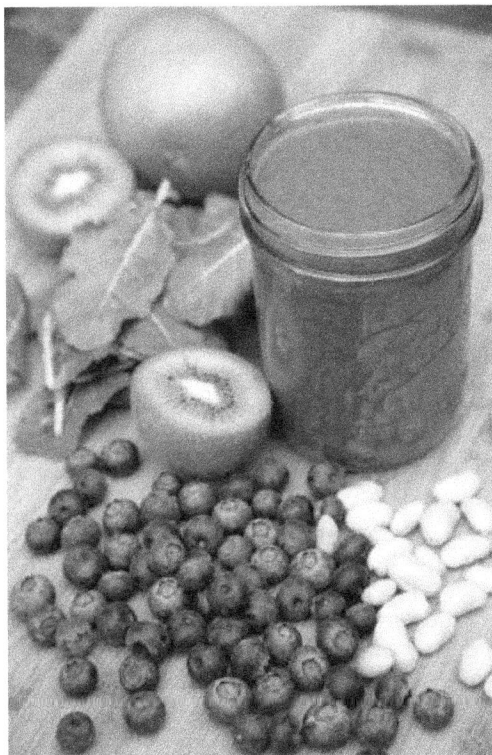

It contains 95 calories in total. You might not love the taste of the recipe but it gives you a lot of anti-oxidants.

Ingredients

- 1 Kiwi, chopped
- 3 tbsp Greek yogurt, fat free
- 1.75 Oz blueberries

Method

1. You can take a bowl, mix all the three ingredients and have a sweet breakfast in morning.

2. You can take the three ingredients in a grinder bowl and grind it. Drink it in a form of smoothie.

Bread with Honey

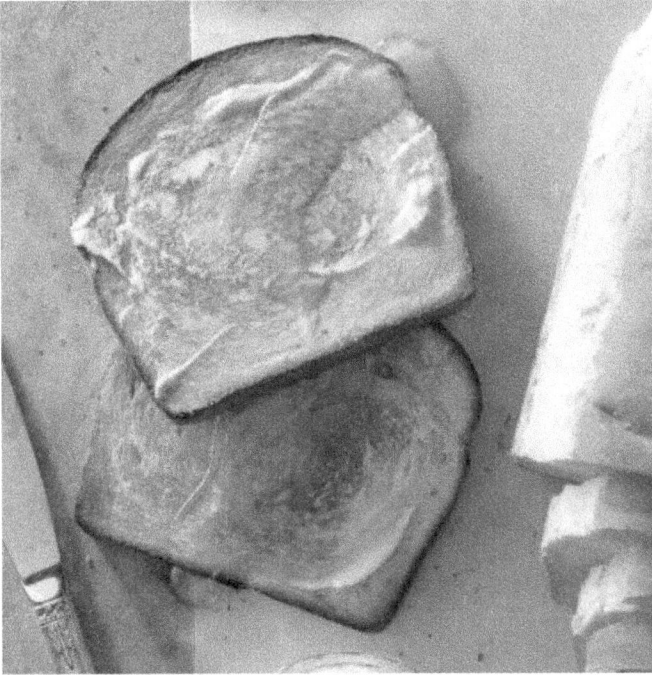

If you need a break of sweet in between your diet plan then you can pour some honey on a slice of bread and enjoy a perfect combination of soft bread with light honey. The recipe contains a total of 95 calories.

Ingredients

- 1 slice of wheat bread
- 2 tbsp honey

Method

1. Take the bread slice and apply honey evenly on the slice. Fold the slice from center and have the perfect morning sandwich.

Mushrooms with Eggs

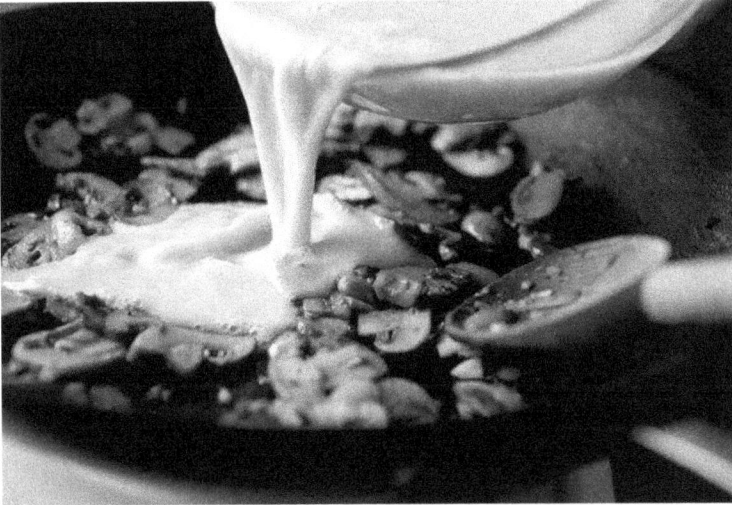

You have to make scrambled eggs but without adding any butter or milk in it. Eggs contain a lot of proteins and you will feel full till afternoon time. Mushrooms add a crispy texture and bulk to the dish. It contains 91 calories.

Ingredients

- 1 medium size egg
- 100 grams Chopped mushroom

Method

1. Take a non-stick pan and pour egg contents in it.

2. Keep stirring the contents till it becomes dry.

3. Add mushroom at the end and have a sumptuous breakfast.

Spinach Omelet

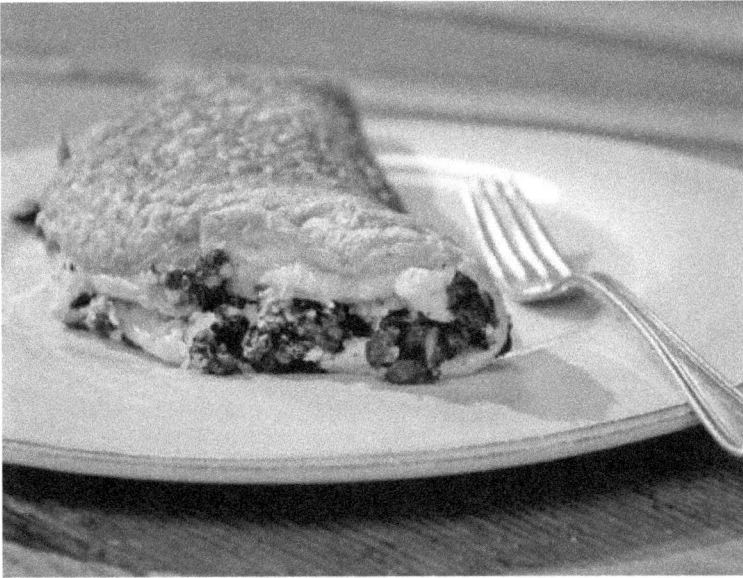

This dish is a perfect way of getting proteins and iron in your morning time. Iron ensures that your hemoglobin level is maintained and protein helps in building your body muscle, which automatically reduces fat.

Ingredients

- 1 egg
- 50 grams chopped spinach
- Salt, pepper and herbs to taste

Method

1. Take a bowl and whisk egg contents in the bowl. Pour the content on griller frying pan and spread the content evenly on pan.

2. Let the omelet cook nicely from bottom and then add chopped spinach from the top. Cook omelet from both the side.

3. Sprinkle some salt, pepper and herbs on top of spinach to add extra flavor to your delicious breakfast.

Fruity Yogurt

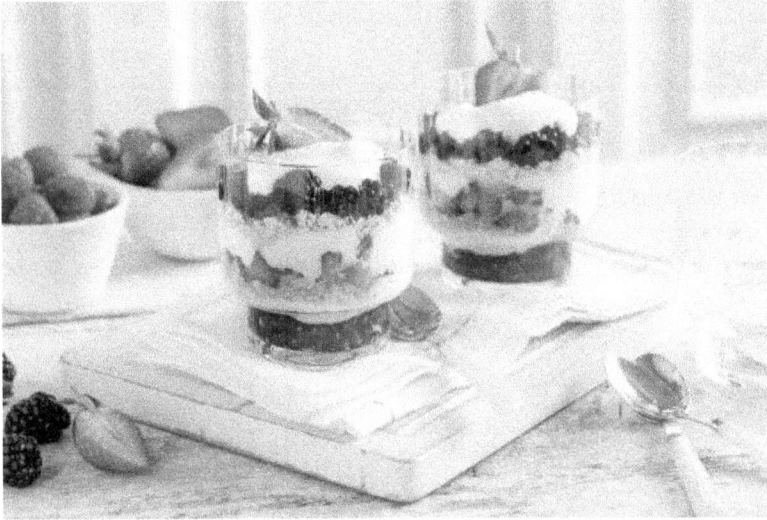

Yogurt contains protein, probiotics, B12, iodine and calcium. All these elements keep you healthy and strong. Iodine, especially, keeps a check on fat around your belly area. It is a great slimming factor. When you combine several mineral rich fruits with it, then this becomes a wholesome dish for you. The dish contains 96 calories.

Ingredients

- 50 grams raspberries
- 50 grams strawberries
- 50 grams blackberries
- 1 apricot
- 3 tbsp Greek yogurt

Method

1. Make thin segments of apricot and chop all the berries that you have.

2. Take a bowl and mix all the ingredients nicely. Enjoy the delicious yogurt.

Honey Porridge

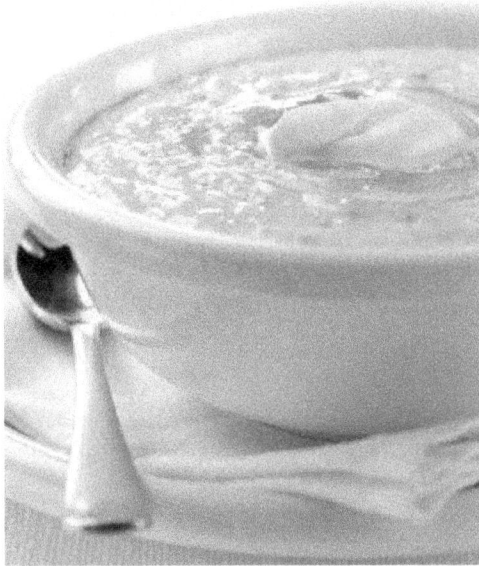

This is one dish that will give some carb boost to your morning. We are making porridge with oats that will keep your full. You can have this recipe when you have a hectic planned morning time. We have also substituted milk with water, which will keep a check on total calorie count.

The dish contains a total of 99 calories. If you are taking less of oats then you can add some nuts and add extra taste to the dish without increasing calorie count.

Ingredients

- ¼ tbsp honey
- 30 grams porridge oats

- ¼ tsp cinnamon
- Water as required

Method

1. Take a bowl and mix porridge oats and honey in the bowl.

2. Mix some water in the bowl to get a good consistency of the dish. Sprinkle cinnamon from top and mix well.

Beans Toast

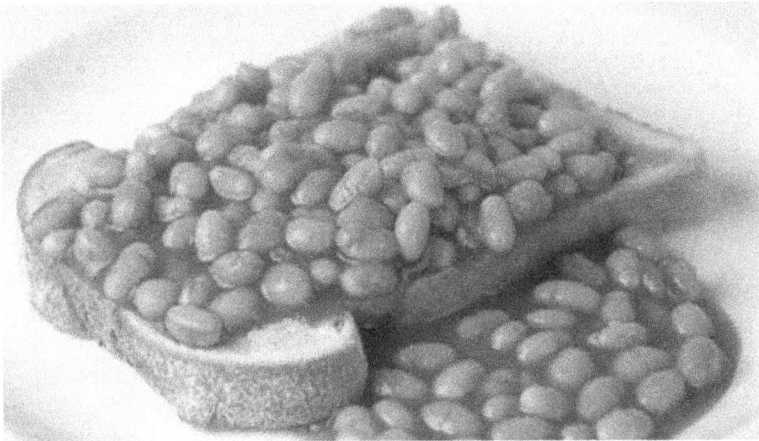

Beans will not increase the calorie count of your breakfast and will add a different taste to your usual routine breakfast. The dish is healthy and is very easy to make. The dish contains a total of 97 calories.

Ingredients

- 1 slice of whole wheat bread
- 50 grams of baked beans

Method

1. Take the bread slice and put it in toaster. Take out bean from a can and heat it in microwave.

2. Apply bean on top of toast and have a delicious breakfast.

Ham Omelet

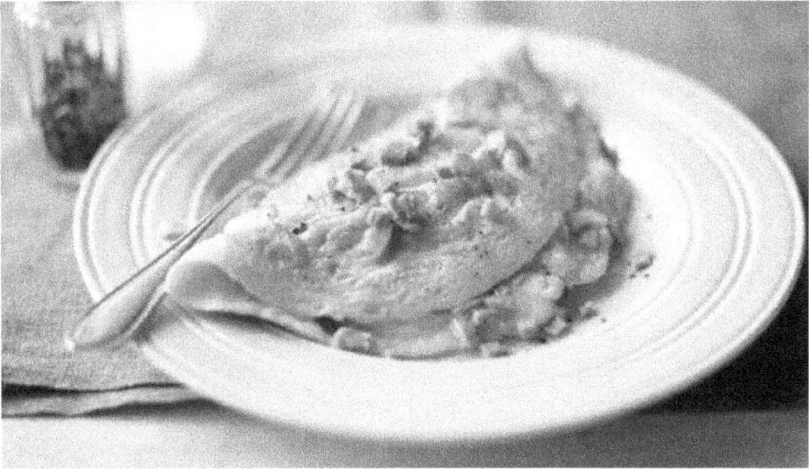

This dish will make you happy because we have a perfect combination of ham and egg in breakfast for you. This is a dish full of proteins and will keep a smile on your face for the whole day long. This dish contains a total of 97 calories.

Ingredients

- 1 egg
- 1 thin ham slice
- Salt and pepper to taste

Method

1. Take a bowl and whisk egg contents properly. Take the ham slice and chop it finely.

2. Take a frying pan and pour whisked egg on the pan. Spread chopped ham evenly on omelet.

3. Sprinkle salt and pepper according to your taste and have a fulfilling breakfast.

Enjoying this book?

Check out my other best sellers!

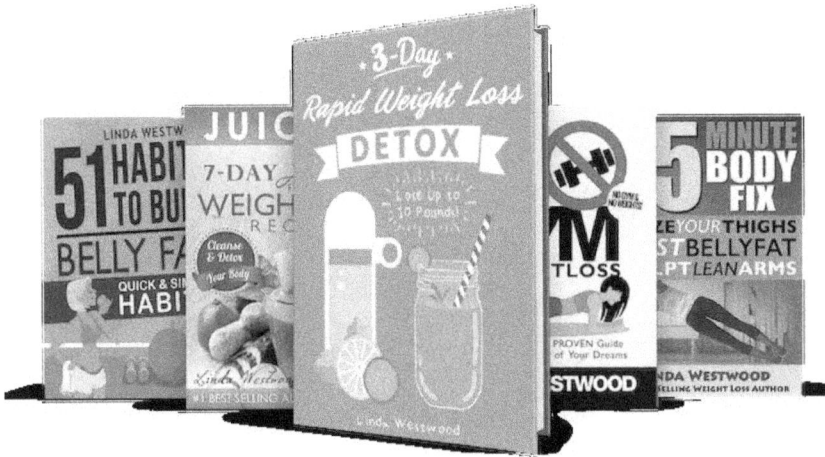

Get your next book on sale here:

TopFitnessAdvice.com/go/books

Chapter 6

2 Days Fasting Recipes for Lunch and Dinner

Controlling your calorie intake during lunch time becomes a bit difficult. It is mid-day and you are basically exhausted with your morning chores. You feel like enjoying a delicious meal without worrying about calorie intake.

We have some good recipes for you that will ensure that your lunch is delicious, you feel full and your calorie intake is below 200 calories, as required under your 5:2 diet plan.

You can have soups, salads and even potatoes; just ensure you take right quantity in right form.

Once again, thank you for reading this book, and I hope you're getting a lot of valuable information. I would greatly appreciate it if you could take 30 seconds to leave me a review for this book on Amazon.com.

Leek Soup with Saffron Twist

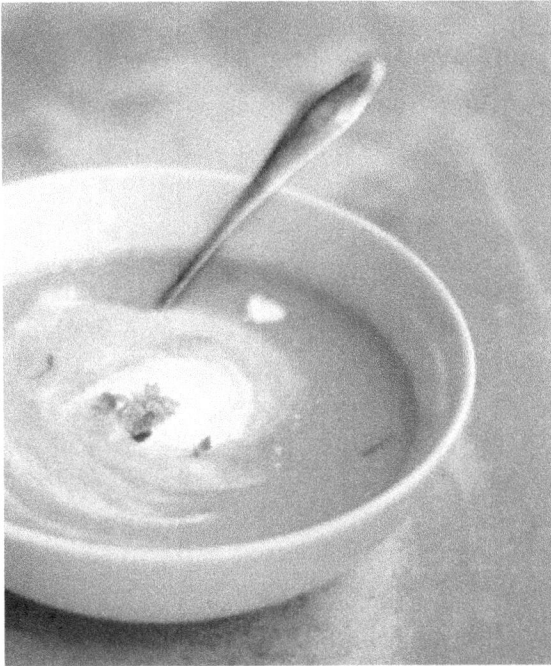

This soup recipe is perfect for your lunch time. It is tasty, crunchy and full of proteins. You can pack it in your lunch box or even store it in freezer for future use. You can have this soup with a crunchy bread toast, but just keep your calories on check. This soup contains a total of 134 calories.

Ingredients

- 100 grams leek
- ¼ cup chopped onion
- 8 grams butter
- ¼ vegetable stock cubes
- 70 grams peeled and chopped potato

- 25 grams peas
- Oil for frying
- A pinch of saffron
- 1/4tbsp flour
- ¼ egg white

Method

1. Take a pan and heat oil in it. Fry onions in the pan for about 10 minutes and add 90 grams sliced leek in the pan.

2. Pour ¼ liters of water in this pan and bring it to boil. Add vegetable stock cube and potato in the pan, and cook the ingredients for about 10 minutes.

3. Add peas and cook all the ingredients for 10 minutes.

4. Take another bowl, whisk egg white, flour and saffron in the bowl. Make a thick batter from this.

5. Cut 10 grams left out leeks into rings and dip them into the flour batter. Cook leek rings on a dry frying pan. Take soup in a bowl and garnish it with leek rings.

Colorful Cabbage Salad

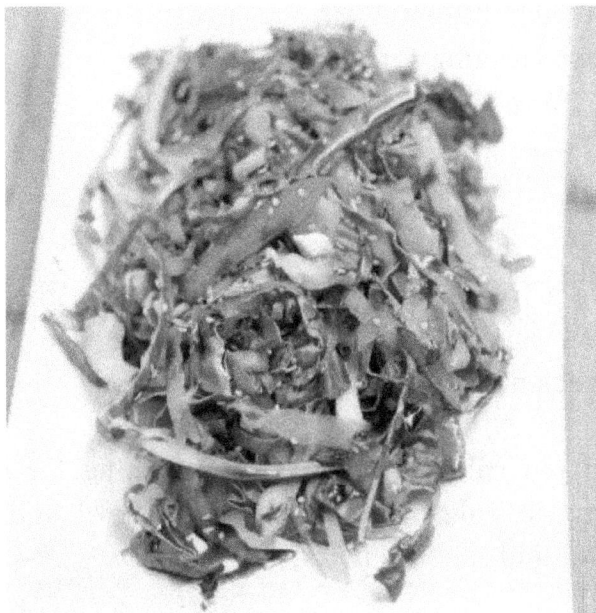

This salad recipe is perfect for a light lunch. The recipe also contains pumpkin seeds which adds a protein punch to the recipe. Other seasoning like fennel and mustard adds a different flavor to the whole recipe. The dish contains 129 calories in total.

Ingredients

- ½ tbs sunflower oil
- ¼ red onion sliced
- 50 grams shredded red cabbage
- 30 grams pointed cabbage
- ¼ small grated carrot
- 1 tsp toasted pumpkin seeds

- ¼ cup parsley
- 1/4tsp wholegrain mustard
- A pinch of brown sugar
- 1/4tsp balsamic vinegar
- 1 tsp olive oil

Method

1. Take a frying pan and heat some oil in the pan. Add onion and fennel in the pan and cook both the ingredients for 2 minutes.

2. Add red cabbage and cook everything for another 3 minutes. Take the contents in a bowl and add raw carrot and cabbage in the bowl.

3. Take another bowl and whisk mustard, pumpkin seeds, olive oil, sugar, vinegar and parsley nicely. Serve the seasoning on the cabbage salad and have a nice lunch.

Steak and Orange Salad

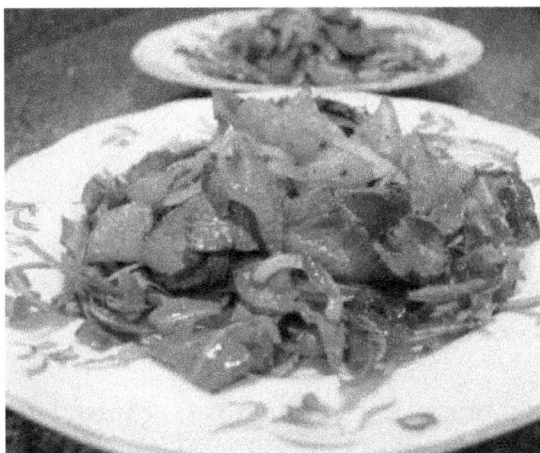

You can make this tender and tangy salad within 30 minutes. This is a perfect recipe for a sunny afternoon, with a hectic evening schedule. You can have this salad individually or can side it with a whole wheat bread slice. This dish contains 179 calories.

Ingredients

- 1.5 tbsp olive oil
- 40 grams sirloin steak, pieces
- ¼ orange segment
- ¼ orange juice
- ½ tbsp sherry vinegar
- ½ tsp mustard
- 2 wedges of onion
- ½ chicory cut into 2 pieces length wise

Method

1. Take steak pieces and rub oil on both the sides of each piece. Take a fry pan and cook all steak pieces on both the sides for about 2 minutes.

2. Wrap all the pieces in a foil and set it aside. Take another pan and boil orange juice in it till it is reduced till half. Add vinegar, mustard and ½ tsp of oil in the orange juice.

3. Add red onion in the oil and cook it till becomes brown in color. Mix all the ingredients in the orange sauce and serve it on plate with red chicory as garnishing.

Chicken Pitta

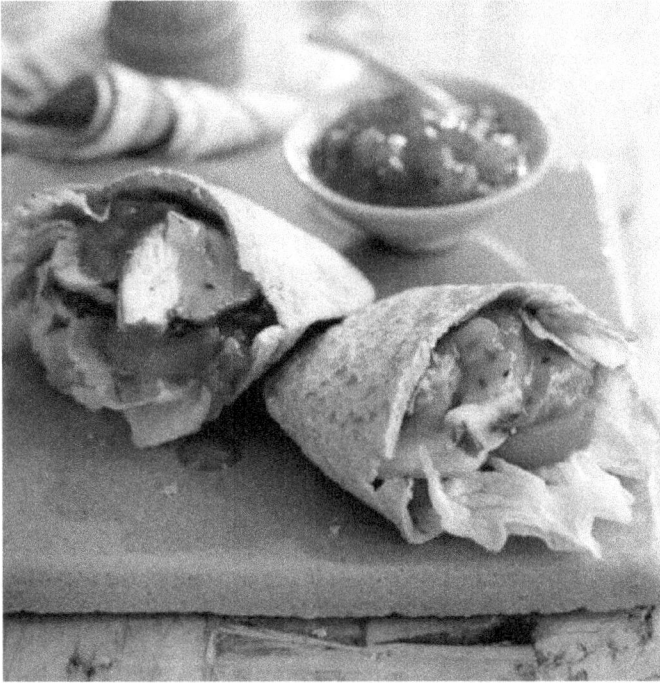

Chicken pitta is a delicious dish that is perfect for a weekend family get together. Even kids love this delicious recipe for their lunch box. Also, you will consume only 162 calories in one chicken pitta serving.

Ingredients

- ½ tbsp natural yogurt
- ½ tsp tomato puree
- ½ tsp curry paste
- 40 grams chicken strips
- 1/4tsp vegetable oil

- 1 pita bread
- 1 tbsp shredded lettuce
- 1 Cherry tomato

Method

1. Take a bowl and mix yogurt, curry paste and tomato puree in it. Toss chicken pieces in the bowl and cover all sides of chicken with paste. Cover chicken and put it in freeze for about 15 minutes.

2. Take a non-stick pan and heat oil in the pan. Cook marinated chicken pieces in the pan for about 8 minutes but ensure chicken piece is still juicy.

3. Take pitta bread and open it. Fill pitta bread with shredded lettuce and chicken pieces in it. Top pitta bread with cherry tomatoes and serve it hot.

Chapter 7

5 Days Fasting Recipes

In the earlier recipes you get to know what all you can have in 2 days of fasting. In this section we will give you recipes that you can have in rest 5 days where you are supposed to have about below 2000 calories per day (2500 for men).

We will give you recipes that are healthy and tasty. You will be amazed to know that we have recipes like pasta and meatballs in store for you. It is not necessary to always have soups and salads when you are on a diet.

I hope that you are enjoying this book so far, and if you could spare 30 seconds, I would greatly appreciate you leaving a review on Amazon.com.

Fish Filo Pastry

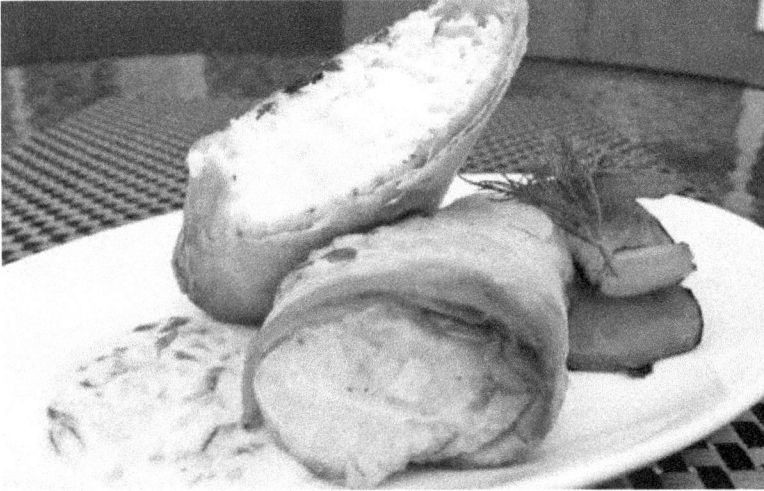

With fish you can get a lot of iodine and remain healthy. The dish contains 463 calories.

Ingredients

- 2 filo pastry sheets
- 2tbsp chopped onion
- 1/2 small bay leaf
- 80ml fish stock
- 12ml white wine
- 120 grams mixed fish like salmon, scallop and raw prawn
- 8 grams plain flour
- 12grams butter
- 25ml fresh cream
- 1tsp lemon zest

- 1 tbsp chopped parsley
- 1 small deseeded and quartered tomato
- Salt and pepper as per taste

Method

1. Take a pan, add stock, wine, bay leaf and onion in it and boil all contents for about 5 minutes. Add large pieces of fish first and add other small pieces after 2 minutes and cook all the content for about 3 more minutes.

2. Take pieces of fish out from the pan and out it in a baking tray. Reheat all the drippings and reduce it will 600 ml and remove bay leaf from it.

3. Take a bowl and mix half of butter and flour in the bowl and make a paste out of it.

4. Add small spoons of mixture in the dripping pan and make a sauce after heating it for 2 minutes. Add cream, lemon zest, parsley, tomato puree, tomato and seasoning in the pan, and at last add fish.

5. Take a filo pastry and brush butter on top of it. Add the sauce and add another sheet on the top with edges tugged in. Bake this dish for 25 minutes at 200 degrees C and serve it hot.

Adding filo pastry in your fish dish will give it that special and crunchy twist.

Chili Meatballs

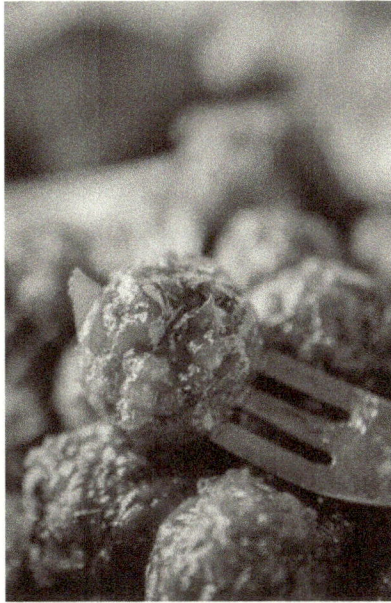

It is always good to have some chili food when you are on a diet plan. At first, they increase the heat within your body which increases the burning down of fat. Secondly, it brings a good change to your usual dull food routine. This dish contains a total of 371 calories.

Ingredients

- 125 grams beef chunks
- 8 grams chili con spice mix
- 1/2 grated small onion
- Cooking spray
- ¼ small chili sliced
- 1 tsp tomato puree

- 200 grams chopped tomato
- 40 ml beef stock
- 100 grams black been
- Salt and pepper as per taste

Method

1. Take a bowl and mix beef, chili mix and onion in it and make 6 balls from the mixture.

2. Take a pan and spray some cooking oil in it and fry all the 6 balls from all the sides for about 10 minutes.

3. Take another pan and heat some cooking oil in it. Add chili, rest of the spice mix and tomato puree and cook for about 1 minute.

4. Add stock and tomatoes to the pan and cook over low flame for 10 minutes.

5. Add meatballs and beans in this pan and cook for another 5 minutes till the sauce becomes thicker. You can serve hot meat balls with some brown rice and enjoy your fiesta.

Chicken Pasta

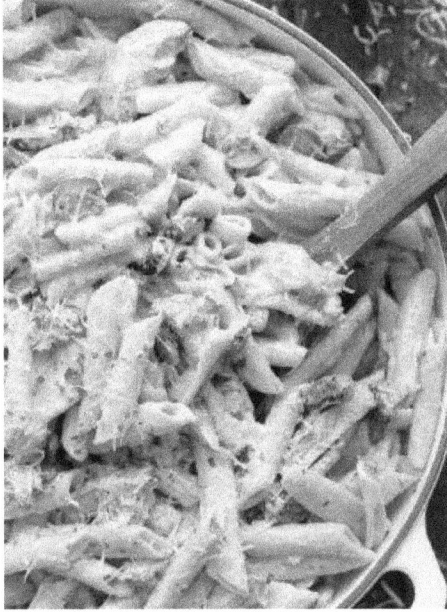

It is an easy dish and you can treat your family with a low calorie yet delicious dish. The dish contains a total of 426 calories.

Ingredients

- 85 grams pasta
- 45 grams peas
- 45 grams cooked chicken chunks
- ½ tsp cream
- 1 tbsp chopped parsley
- Salt and pepper as per taste

Method

1. Cook pasta as per instructed in the packet. Just before the pasta is fully cooked, 3 minutes before, add peas to the boiling pan.

2. Drain the two ingredients and shift it to a pan. Add chicken, parsley and cream in the pan.

3. Put the pan over medium flame and cook everything for 2 minutes. Sprinkle salt and pepper from the top.

Others who are considering purchasing this book would love to know what you think. If you could spare a few seconds, they would greatly appreciate reading an honest review from you. Simply visit it on Amazon.com.

Cod Nuggets and Wedged Sweet Potato

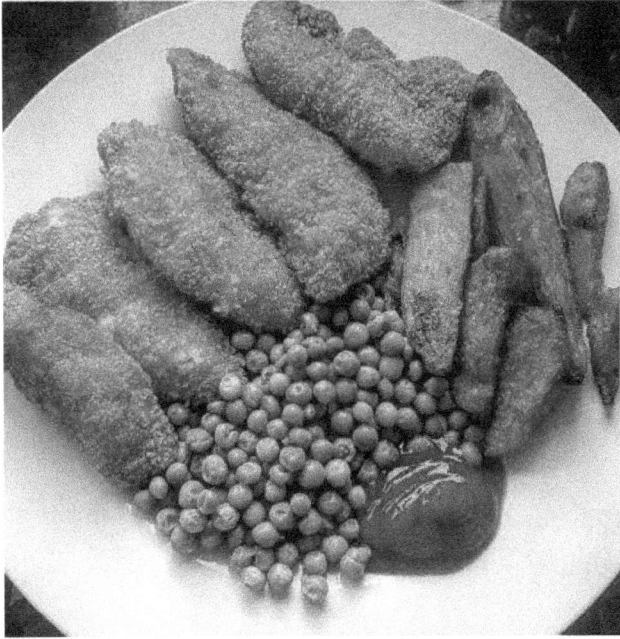

Fish fingers are good for your taste buds as well as for your health. To make this recipe healthier, we have added a flavor of sweet potato chips instead of normal ones. This dish has a total of 480 calories.

Ingredients

- 1 cod filled chunked
- 1/2tbsp plain flour
- ½ egg beaten
- 25 grams wheat bread crumbs
- 8ml olive oil

- ½ sweet potato cut into wedges
- 4ml honey
- Sunflower oil
- Sour cream

Method

1. Take a piece of cod, cover it in flour, dip it in beaten egg and then make a final coat of bread crumbs. Cover all the pieces and put it in freeze for about 20 minutes.

2. Take a roasting tin and heat olive oil for about 4 minutes and add sweet potatoes in it. Roast the cod in tin for about 20 minutes by turning it up and down.

3. Brush the pieces with honey and cook it till it becomes tender in oven for about 10 minutes.

4. Take a fry pan and heat sunflower oil in it. Fry fish pieces on all the sides in the pan for about 3 minutes.

5. Drain oil with the help of tissue paper and serve it with sweet potato wedges.

Thai Noodles

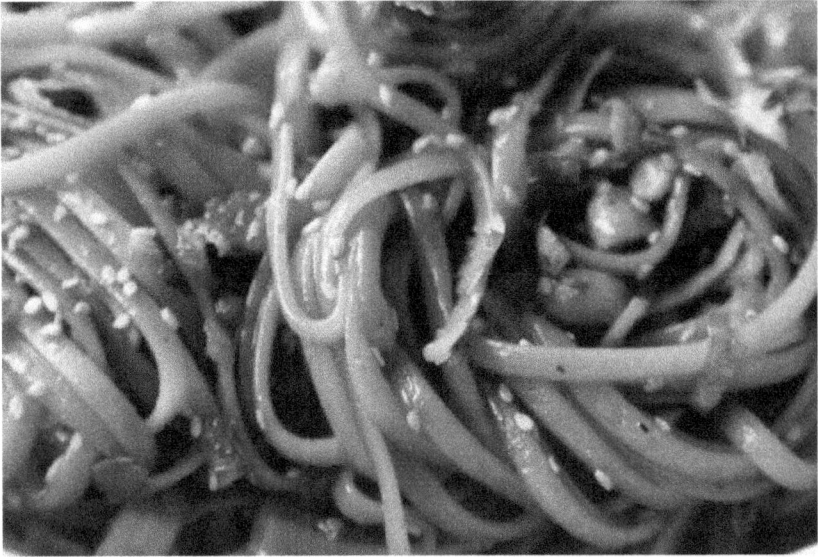

There is something special about all the Thai dishes. The special Thai ingredients give a very different taste to normal noodles. All the ingredients are readily available because of which you can make this dish is a very less time. This dish contains a total of 307 calories.

Ingredients

- ¾ tbsp Thai curry paste
- 90-gram Butternut squash and sweet potato
- 55ml coconut milk
- ½ vegetable stock cubes
- 34 grams frozen peas
- 50 grams readymade noodles
- 1/3rd pak choi head

- Basil leaves
- Red chili

Method

1. Take a large pan and add Thai paste and butternut sweet potato squash in the pan. Stir fry all the contents for about 2 minutes on medium heat.

2. Add coconut milk and hot water in the pan. Add stock cubes in the pan and simmer all the contents for about 15 minutes till all the vegetables get tender.

3. Add peas to the pan, add noodles and let all the ingredients simmer for about 2 minutes. Take pak choi and pour hot water in it. Serve curry in bowls along with pak choi.

Chapter 8

Powerful Diet Plans That Work

Your body needs calories on a daily basis, which you get from the food you take on a daily basis. When the amount of calorie that your body needs exceeds the amount you intake, then your body starts using the stored energy. This stored energy is fats. If your body suffers from this deficiency for a long time, then you start reducing your body weight and fat. This is however, a basic explanation.

There are two sources of energy for body, on a daily basis; carbohydrates and fats. For some, metabolism works perfectly well when we limit their calorie intake. For some, the count of calorie does not matter because their body energy depends heavily on the carbohydrate levels. When their carbohydrate intake is decreased, they automatically reduce weight. Atkins weight plan follow the second technique.

There is another diet plan, 7 days diet plan, which produces great effect on human body. In this you are supposed to eat a specific diet for each day for a total of seven days, where you get to eat a mixture of fruits, salads, milk and rice.

In this plan, basically you reduce the intake of carbohydrate and give a continuous supply of protein to your body. This protein goes into building muscle in your body, which in turn decreases the stored fat content of your body. Also, you cleanse your body over 7 days with a continuous supply of fibers and minerals, which again helps in decreasing fat content of body.

You should know what kind of plan will suit your body and you should accordingly follow a plan. To make your 5:2 diet work well we are giving you some truly exciting recipes with the help of which you will not even feel that you are on a diet plan, and yet it will show results on your body.

I hope you have learned something from this book so far and would greatly appreciate it if you could leave an honest review on Amazon.com.

Discover Scientifically-Proven "Shortcuts" & "Hacks" to Lose Weight FASTER (With Very Little Effort)

For this month only, you can get Linda's best-selling & most popular book absolutely free – *Weight Loss Secrets You NEED to Know.*

Get Your FREE Copy Here:

TopFitnessAdvice.com/Bonus

Discover scientifically-proven tips to help you lose weight faster and easier than ever before. With this book, readers were able to improve their weight loss results and fitness levels. So, it's highly recommended that you get this book, especially while it's free!

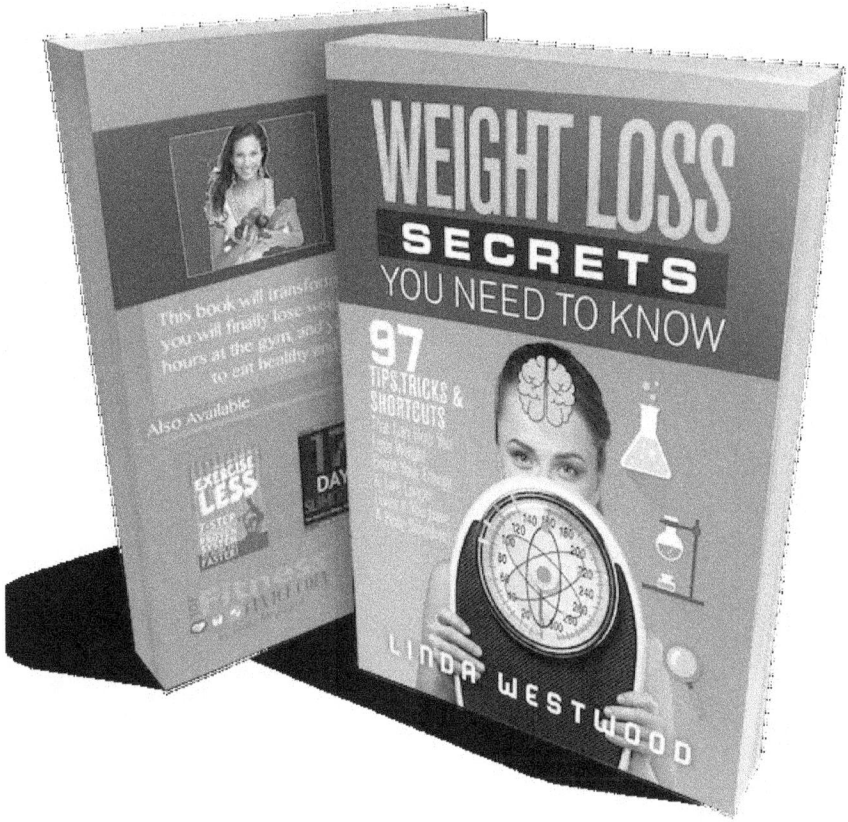

Get Your FREE Copy Here:

TopFitnessAdvice.com/Bonus

Final Words

I would like to thank you for purchasing my book and I hope I have been able to help you and educate you on something new.

If you have enjoyed this book and would like to share your positive thoughts, could you please take 30 seconds of your time to go back and give me a review on my Amazon book page.

I greatly appreciate seeing these reviews because it helps me share my hard work.

You can leave me a review on Amazon.com.

Again, thank you and I wish you all the best!

Enjoying this book?

Check out my other best sellers!

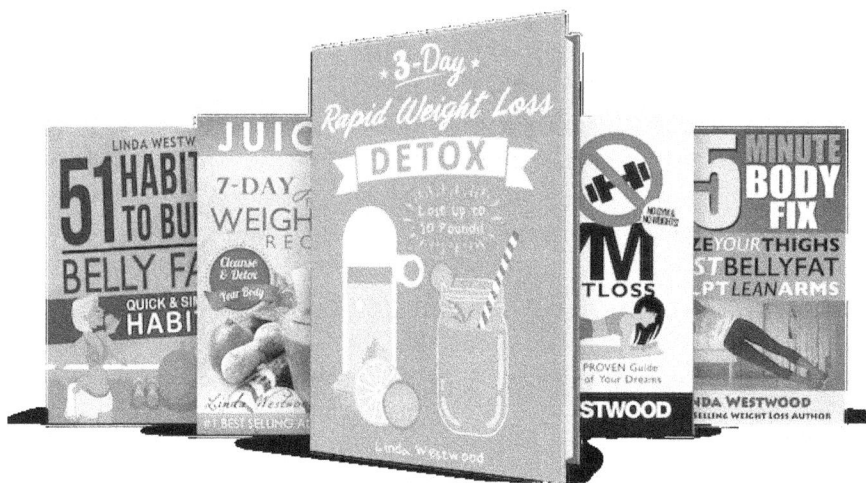

Get your next book on sale here:

TopFitnessAdvice.com/go/books

.

www.ingramcontent.com/pod-product-compliance
Lightning Source LLC
Chambersburg PA
CBHW031209020426
42333CB00013B/856